WEIGHT LOSS GUIDE: Discover healthy eating habits and how to manage weight.

Chanel C. Jones

Table Of Contents

Negative calorie preloading
Sleep Enhancement
Stress Hormone Relief
Wall off Calories

The state of nutrition

Nutrition is the process by which the body takes in and uses food to sustain itself. It is an essential aspect of maintaining good health, as the nutrients in food provide the energy and building blocks the body needs to function properly.

There are several key nutrients that the body needs in order to stay healthy. These include carbohydrates, proteins, fats, vitamins, and minerals. Each of these nutrients plays a specific role in the body, and it is important to consume a balanced diet that includes a variety of these nutrients in order to meet the body's needs.

Carbohydrates are the body's primary source of energy, and they are found in foods like grains, fruits, and vegetables. Proteins are essential for building and repairing tissues, and they are found in foods like meat, fish, dairy products, and beans. Fats are important for energy storage and insulation, and they are found in foods like oils, nuts, and avocados. Vitamins and minerals are essential for various functions in the body, and they are found in a wide range of foods including fruits, vegetables, grains, and dairy products.

Maintaining good nutrition involves consuming a balanced diet that includes a variety of different types of foods. It is also important to pay attention to portion sizes and to limit the intake of unhealthy or processed foods that are high in calories, sugar, and unhealthy fats.

Industrial Nutrition Advice

Industrial nutrition refers to the science of how nutrition impacts the health and performance of people who work in industrial settings. Industrial nutrition advice typically focuses on the nutritional needs of people who work in physically demanding jobs or who are exposed to hazardous substances on a regular basis.

Some key considerations in industrial nutrition advice include:

Energy needs: People who work in physically demanding jobs or who work long hours may have higher energy needs than those who are sedentary. Industrial nutrition advice may include recommendations for foods that are high in energy-providing nutrients, such as carbohydrates and fats.

Hydration: Dehydration can impact performance and safety on the job. Industrial nutrition advice may include recommendations for staying hydrated, such as drinking plenty of water and electrolyte-rich beverages.

Nutrient needs: Industrial workers may have increased needs for certain nutrients due to the physical demands of their job or exposure to hazardous substances. Industrial nutrition advice may include recommendations for foods that are rich in these nutrients.

Workplace wellness programs: Many industrial companies have wellness programs that include nutrition education and resources for employees. These programs may include information on healthy eating habits, food choices, and ways to maintain good nutrition while working long hours or in physically demanding conditions.

The Foundation of Nutrition

The foundation of nutrition is the intake of a variety of nutrients that the body needs to function properly. These nutrients include carbohydrates, proteins, fats, vitamins, and minerals.

Carbohydrates are the body's primary source of energy, and they are found in foods like grains, fruits, and vegetables. Proteins are essential for building and repairing tissues, and they are found in foods like meat, fish, dairy products, and beans. Fats are important for energy storage and insulation, and they are found in foods like oils, nuts, and avocados. Vitamins and minerals are essential for various functions in the body, and they are found in a wide range of foods including fruits, vegetables, grains, and dairy products.

Maintaining good nutrition involves consuming a balanced diet that includes a variety of different types of foods. It is also important to pay attention to portion sizes and to limit the intake of unhealthy or processed foods that are high in calories, sugar, and unhealthy fats.

In addition to the intake of nutrients, the foundation of nutrition also includes the body's ability to absorb and use those nutrients effectively. This involves the proper functioning of the digestive system, as well as the presence of sufficient enzymes and other substances that help the body break down and use nutrients.

Why you Need to Eat Healthy

Eating a healthy diet is important for maintaining good health and preventing a variety of health problems. Some key reasons to eat healthy include:

Weight management: A healthy diet can help you maintain a healthy weight and reduce the risk of obesity and related health problems such as diabetes, heart disease, and some cancers.

Energy: A healthy diet can provide the energy your body needs to function properly and stay active.

Mental health: A healthy diet can help improve mood and cognitive function and reduce the risk of mental health problems such as depression and anxiety.

Physical health: A healthy diet can help reduce the risk of a variety of physical health problems, including heart disease, stroke, some cancers, and osteoporosis.

Longevity: A healthy diet may help you live a longer, healthier life.

Eating a healthy diet is an important aspect of maintaining good health and preventing a variety of health problems. It is important to consume a balanced diet that includes a variety of different types of foods, pay attention to portion sizes, and limit the intake of unhealthy or processed foods that are high in calories, sugar, and unhealthy fats.

The "Myth" of Healthy Foods

There is often a lot of misinformation and misunderstanding surrounding the concept of "healthy" foods. Some people may believe that certain foods are healthy simply because they are marketed as such, or because they are perceived as being natural or organic. However, it is important to remember that not all foods that are marketed as healthy or natural are actually good for you.

For example, some so-called "healthy" foods may be high in calories, sugar, or unhealthy fats, and may not provide the nutrients the body needs to function properly. In addition, some foods that are marketed as natural or organic may not be grown or processed in a way that is truly healthy or sustainable.

It is important to be aware of these myths and to base your food choices on sound, evidence-based nutrition guidelines rather than marketing claims or perceptions of what is healthy. A healthy diet should include a variety of different types of foods, including whole grains, fruits, vegetables, lean proteins, and healthy fats. It is also important to pay attention to portion sizes and to limit the intake of unhealthy or processed foods that are high in calories, sugar, and unhealthy fats.

What is an Ideal Diet

An ideal diet is one that provides all the nutrients the body needs to function properly and maintain good health. It should include a variety of different types of foods, in the right proportions, and be appropriate for a person's age, sex, weight, and activity level.

An ideal diet should include:

Plenty of fruits and vegetables: These provide essential vitamins, minerals, and fiber.

Whole grains: These provide energy, fiber, and essential nutrients.

Lean proteins: These include foods like chicken, fish, tofu, and beans, and are important for building and repairing tissues.

Healthy fats: These include foods like nuts, seeds, avocados, and olive oil, and are important for energy storage and insulation.

Limited amounts of added sugars and unhealthy fats: These should be consumed in moderation, as they can contribute to weight gain and increase the risk of health problems.

What to Eat to Stay Healthy

Eating a healthy diet is an important aspect of maintaining good health and preventing a variety of health problems. Some general guidelines for what to eat to stay healthy include:

Eat a variety of different types of foods: A healthy diet should include a variety of different types of foods, including whole grains, fruits, vegetables, lean proteins, and healthy fats.

Choose whole, unprocessed foods: These types of foods are generally more nutritious and have fewer additives and preservatives.

Limit added sugars and unhealthy fats: Foods high in added sugars and unhealthy fats, such as saturated and trans fats, should be consumed in moderation, as they can contribute to weight gain and increase the risk of health problems.

Pay attention to portion sizes: It is important to pay attention to how much you are eating, as overconsumption of any type of food can lead to weight gain and other health problems.

Drink plenty of water: Staying hydrated is important for maintaining good health. Aim to drink at least 8 cups of water per day, and more if you are physically active or live in a hot climate.

When to Eat to Stay Healthy
In addition to what you eat, the timing of your meals and snacks can also impact your health. Some general guidelines for when to eat to stay healthy include:

Eat regular meals: Aim to eat at least three main meals per day, with snacks in between if needed. This can help keep your energy levels stable and prevent overeating at meal times.

Don't skip breakfast: Breakfast is an important meal that can help kickstart your metabolism and provide energy for the day.

Avoid eating late at night: Eating late at night can disrupt your sleep and may lead to weight gain. Try to finish your last meal of the day at least a few hours before bedtime.

Don't go too long without eating: Going too long without eating can lead to overeating at the next meal, as well as low energy levels. Try to eat every 3-4 hours to keep your energy levels stable.

Why People get Fat

There are many reasons why people may gain weight or become overweight. Some common reasons include:

Overeating: Consuming more calories than the body needs can lead to weight gain.

Lack of physical activity: Burning fewer calories than you consume can lead to weight gain, particularly if you have a sedentary lifestyle.

Genetics: Certain genetic factors can make it more likely for a person to gain weight or have difficulty losing weight.

Medical conditions: Certain medical conditions, such as hypothyroidism or polycystic ovary syndrome, can lead to weight gain.

Medications: Some medications, such as antidepressants and steroids, can cause weight gain as a side effect.

Stress: High levels of stress can lead to unhealthy eating habits, such as overeating or binge eating, which can contribute to weight gain.

Sleep deprivation: Lack of sleep can affect the hormones that regulate hunger and fullness, leading to weight gain.

The Most Effective Weight Loss Habit

The most effective weight loss habit is consistent, long-term adherence to a healthy diet and regular physical activity. There is no one "magic" habit that will lead to weight loss, and it's important to remember that everyone is different and what works for one person may not work for another. However, here are some habits that can contribute to successful weight loss:

Eating a balanced diet: This means getting enough nutrients from a variety of sources, including fruits, vegetables, whole grains, lean protein, and healthy fats.

Engaging in regular physical activity: Aim for at least 150 minutes of moderate-intensity exercise or 75 minutes of vigorous-intensity exercise per week, as recommended by the Centers for Disease Control and Prevention (CDC).

Monitoring portion sizes: Pay attention to how much you eat, as well as the types and amounts of foods you consume. Using measuring cups or a food scale can help you keep track of portion sizes.

Keeping track of your food intake: Writing down what you eat can help you become more aware of your food choices and identify any unhealthy eating patterns.

Being consistent: It's important to make healthy habits a regular part of your lifestyle, rather than just trying to "diet" for a short period of time. Getting enough sleep: Getting enough sleep is important for weight loss because it helps regulate hunger hormones and can improve your overall energy levels. Aim for 7-9 hours of sleep per night.

Ingredients for the Ideal Weight-loss Diet

The ideal weight-loss diet should be balanced and include a variety of nutrient-dense foods. Some key ingredients to include are:

Fruits and vegetables: These are high in fiber, vitamins, and minerals, and low in calories. Aim for a variety of colors and types to get a range of nutrients.

Lean protein sources: These include chicken, turkey, fish, beans, and tofu. Protein can help keep you feeling full and satisfied, which can help with weight loss.

Whole grains: Choose whole grains like brown rice, quinoa, and oats over refined grains like white rice and pasta. Whole grains are higher in fiber and nutrients.

Healthy fats: These include monounsaturated and polyunsaturated fats, which can be found in foods like avocados, nuts, and olive oil. These fats can help with weight loss and are important for overall health.

Water: Staying hydrated is important for weight loss and overall health. Aim for at least 8 cups of water per day.

Weight-loss Boosters

Weight loss boosters are techniques or strategies that can help to accelerate weight loss or increase the effectiveness of a weight loss program. Here are some examples of weight loss boosters:

Incorporating high-intensity interval training (HIIT) into your exercise routine: HIIT is a type of exercise that involves short bursts of intense activity followed by periods of rest. It has been shown to be effective for weight loss and can help to boost metabolism.

Adding resistance training to your workout routine: Resistance training, also known as strength training, involves using weights or other resistance to build muscle mass. This can help to increase metabolism and burn more calories, even at rest.

Eating protein-rich foods: Protein can help to keep you feeling full and satisfied, which may make it easier to stick to a calorie-controlled diet. It can also help to preserve muscle mass during weight loss, which can help to maintain metabolism.

Getting enough sleep: Poor sleep can disrupt hormone levels and metabolism, which can make it harder to lose weight. Aim for 7-9 hours of sleep per night to support weight loss efforts.

Managing stress: Chronic stress can lead to weight gain, so finding healthy ways to manage stress, such as through exercise, meditation, or therapy, can be helpful for weight loss.

Drinking plenty of water: Staying hydrated can help to keep you feeling full and can also support healthy digestion.

Benefits of Eating Right

Eating a healthy and balanced diet has a number of benefits for overall health and well-being. Here are some specific benefits of eating right:

Weight management: A healthy diet can help you maintain a healthy weight or lose weight if needed. This is because eating a diet that is high in nutrient-dense foods and low in calories can help you feel full and satisfied while still maintaining a calorie deficit.

Improved digestion: A healthy diet that is high in fiber can help to support healthy digestion and prevent constipation.

Increased energy: Eating a diet that is rich in nutrients, such as fruits, vegetables, and whole grains, can help to provide sustained energy throughout the day.

Stronger immune system: A healthy diet that is high in fruits, vegetables, and other plant-based foods can help to support a strong immune system. These foods are rich in antioxidants and other nutrients that can help to protect against illness and disease.

Better mental health: There is some evidence to suggest that a healthy diet can help to improve mood and reduce the risk of mental health conditions such as depression and anxiety.

Lower risk of chronic diseases: Eating a healthy diet can help to reduce the risk of developing chronic diseases such as heart disease, diabetes, and certain types of cancer.

Losing Weight by Eating Right

There are several ways that eating right can help with weight loss:

Focus on nutrient-dense, low-calorie foods: Choose foods that are high in nutrients and low in calories, such as fruits, vegetables, lean proteins, and whole grains. These foods can help to keep you feeling full and satisfied while still allowing you to maintain a calorie deficit, which is necessary for weight loss.

Limit added sugars and unhealthy fats: Foods that are high in added sugars and unhealthy fats, such as sugar-sweetened beverages, fast food, and baked goods, are often high in calories and low in nutrients. Limiting these foods can help to reduce calorie intake and support weight loss.

Eat regularly and don't skip meals: Skipping meals or going long periods without eating can lead to overeating later on, which can make it harder to maintain a calorie deficit. Instead, aim to eat regular, balanced meals throughout the day to help control appetite and cravings.

Stay hydrated: Drinking plenty of water can help to keep you feeling full and satisfied, which can make it easier to stick to a calorie-controlled diet.

Eat slowly and mindfully: Pay attention to your food as you eat and take your time to enjoy each bite. This can help you to feel satisfied with smaller portions and can also help to prevent overeating.

Eating Right and Managing your Life.

Eating a healthy diet and managing your life can be challenging, but it is an important part of maintaining good physical and mental health. Here are some tips to help you eat right and manage your life:

Plan ahead: Take the time to plan your meals and snacks for the week. This will help you make healthier choices and avoid impulse eating. You can also prepare meals in advance to save time and reduce stress.

Eat a variety of foods: To get all the nutrients your body needs, it is important to eat a variety of foods from all food groups. This includes fruits, vegetables, whole grains, protein sources such as meat, poultry, fish, beans, and nuts, and healthy fats.

Practice portion control: It is important to pay attention to portion sizes to ensure that you are not consuming too many calories. Using smaller plates and measuring cups can help you practice portion control.

Stay hydrated: Drinking enough water is important for maintaining good health. Aim to drink at least 8 cups of water per day.

Get enough sleep: Getting enough sleep is important for both physical and mental health. Aim for 7-9 hours of sleep per night.

Exercise regularly: Regular physical activity can help you maintain a healthy weight, reduce stress, and improve your overall health. Aim for at least 30 minutes of moderate-intensity activity per day.

Manage stress: Chronic stress can have negative effects on your physical and mental health. Finding healthy ways to manage stress, such as through exercise, meditation, or talking to a trusted friend or family member, can help you maintain good overall health.

Exercise Tweaks

There are many ways you can make small changes to your exercise routine to improve its effectiveness and keep it interesting. Here are a few ideas:

Mix up your workouts: Instead of doing the same workout every day, try switching things up by adding new exercises or activities to your routine. This will help prevent boredom and keep your muscles challenged.

Increase intensity: If you find that your workouts are no longer challenging, try increasing the intensity. This can be done by increasing the weight you use, doing more reps, or increasing the speed or intensity of your workouts.

Add variety: Incorporating different types of exercise into your routine, such as strength training, cardio, or yoga, can help keep things interesting and provide a full-body workout.

Take breaks: It's important to allow your body time to rest and recover between workouts. Taking a day or two off each week can help prevent burnout and allow your muscles to recover.

Find a workout buddy: Working out with a friend or family member can make exercise more fun and help keep you motivated.

By making small tweaks to your exercise routine, you can keep your workouts interesting and effective.

Fat burners

Fat burners are supplements that are claimed to help you lose weight by increasing your metabolism and reducing your appetite. There is limited scientific evidence to support the effectiveness of fat burners, and they may have potential side effects.

Exercise is a more reliable and healthy way to lose weight and burn fat. A combination of cardiovascular exercise (such as running, cycling, or swimming) and strength training can help you achieve your weight loss and fat loss goals. Cardiovascular exercise can help you burn calories and fat, while strength training can help you build lean muscle mass, which can increase your metabolism and help you burn more calories even at rest.

It's important to remember that losing weight and burning fat requires a combination of diet and exercise. No supplement or exercise alone can help you lose weight if you are not also following a healthy diet and getting enough sleep. It's also important to speak with a healthcare professional before starting any new exercise program or taking any supplements.

Intermittent Fasting

Intermittent fasting is an eating pattern that involves cycling between periods of fasting and eating. The goal of intermittent fasting is to reduce overall calorie intake, which may lead to weight loss and other potential health benefits. There are several different methods of intermittent fasting, including:

The 16/8 method: This involves fasting for 16 hours and eating during an 8-hour window. For example, you might eat all of your meals between 12 PM and 8 PM and then fast until 12 PM the next day.

The 5:2 diet: This involves eating normally for 5 days and restricting calories to 500-600 per day for the other 2 nonconsecutive days.

Alternate-day fasting: This involves alternating between days of eating normally and days of restricted calorie intake.

Intermittent fasting may have various health benefits, such as weight loss, improved insulin sensitivity, and reduced inflammation.

It's also important to remember that intermittent fasting is not a substitute for a healthy diet. While it may be an effective tool for weight loss, it's important to choose nutrient-dense foods during your eating periods to support overall health.

Hydration

Hydration is the process of replenishing the fluids in your body. It is important to stay hydrated because your body needs an adequate supply of fluids to function properly. Water makes up a large part of your body and is essential for maintaining the balance of bodily fluids, regulating body temperature, and supporting various bodily functions.

There are a few signs that you may not be drinking enough water, including feeling thirsty, having a dry mouth, feeling tired, and having infrequent or dark urine. To ensure that you are getting enough water, aim to drink at least 8 cups (64 ounces) of water per day. You can also get fluids from other beverages and foods, such as milk, juice, and fruits and vegetables with a high water content.

In addition to drinking water, it is also important to pay attention to your body's thirst signals and drink water when you feel thirsty. It is also a good idea to carry a water bottle with you throughout the day to help you stay hydrated.

Meal Frequency

Eating frequency, or how often you eat, can affect weight loss. Some people find it helpful to eat smaller, more frequent meals throughout the day, while others prefer to eat larger, less frequent meals. There is no one-size-fits-all approach to meal frequency and weight loss, and the right approach for you may depend on your individual needs, preferences, and lifestyle.

There are a few factors to consider when it comes to meal frequency and weight loss:

Calorie intake: To lose weight, you need to create a calorie deficit by burning more calories than you consume. Regardless of how often you eat, it's important to pay attention to the total number of calories you consume each day.

Satiety: Some people find that eating smaller, more frequent meals helps them feel full and satisfied, which can be helpful for weight loss.

Blood sugar control: Eating smaller, more frequent meals may help keep blood sugar levels stable, which can be beneficial for weight loss.

Hunger and cravings: If you tend to feel hungry or have cravings between meals, eating more frequently may help keep these feelings at bay.

Ultimately, the best approach to meal frequency and weight loss is one that works for you and helps you maintain a healthy, calorie-controlled diet. It's important to listen to your body's hunger and fullness cues and choose an eating pattern that feels sustainable for you.

Metabolic Boosters

Metabolic boosters are substances or practices that are believed to increase the rate at which the body burns calories, or metabolism. Some people may use metabolic boosters in an attempt to lose weight or improve athletic performance.

There are a few different types of metabolic boosters that people may use, including:

Thermogenic supplements: These are dietary supplements that are believed to increase the body's metabolic rate by generating heat. Some examples include caffeine, green tea extract, and capsaicin (found in chili peppers).

High-intensity interval training (HIIT): This type of exercise involves short bursts of intense activity followed by periods of rest. HIIT has been shown to be effective at increasing metabolic rate, both during and after exercise.

Strength training: Resistance training (such as lifting weights) has been shown to increase metabolic rate, as the body burns more calories to repair and rebuild muscle tissue after a workout.

Negative calorie preloading

There is no scientific evidence to support the concept of "negative calorie preloading," which refers to the idea that certain foods require more calories to digest than they contain, resulting in a net negative caloric intake when consumed. All foods have calories, and the body requires a certain number of calories to function properly. While some foods may have fewer calories than others, it is not possible for a food to have negative calories.

It is true that some foods, such as certain fruits and vegetables, are low in calories and can be part of a healthy weight loss plan. However, these foods should not be relied upon as a means of "preloading" or "offsetting" the calories from other, more caloric foods. The best way to manage weight and maintain a healthy diet is to focus on eating a variety of nutritious foods in moderation, getting regular physical activity, and managing stress and other factors that can affect appetite and food choices.

Sleep Enhancement

Getting a good night's sleep is essential for overall health and well-being. Adequate sleep helps to support physical and mental health, as well as cognitive function, mood, and quality of life. There are several ways to enhance sleep, including:

Establishing a consistent sleep schedule: Try to go to bed and wake up at the same time every day, even on weekends. This can help regulate your body's natural sleep-wake cycle.

Creating a sleep-friendly environment: Keep your bedroom dark, cool, and quiet, and remove electronics and other distractions. A comfortable bed and pillows can also help improve sleep quality.

Practicing relaxation techniques: Try relaxation techniques such as deep breathing, meditation, or yoga before bedtime to help calm the mind and prepare the body for sleep.

Avoiding stimulating activities before bed: Avoid consuming caffeine, alcohol, and heavy meals close to bedtime, as these can interfere with sleep. It is also a good idea to avoid screen time (e.g., watching TV, using a computer) for at least an hour before bed, as the blue light emitted by screens can disrupt the body's natural sleep-wake cycle.

Exercising regularly: Regular physical activity can help improve sleep quality, but it is important to avoid vigorous exercise close to bedtime, as it can stimulate the body and make it harder to fall asleep.

Stress Hormone Relief

There are several ways to help reduce stress and the production of stress hormones in the body:

Exercise: Physical activity can help reduce stress and improve overall physical and mental health.

Practice relaxation techniques: Techniques such as deep breathing, meditation, or yoga can help calm the mind and reduce stress.

Get enough sleep: Adequate sleep is important for managing stress and maintaining overall health and well-being.

Eat a healthy diet: A diet rich in fruits, vegetables, and other nutrients can help support overall health and reduce stress.

Stay hydrated: Drinking enough water can help keep the body and mind functioning optimally and reduce stress.

Connect with others: Social support can be an important source of comfort and can help reduce stress.

Take breaks: Taking breaks from work and other responsibilities can help reduce stress and improve overall well-being.

Seek support: If stress becomes overwhelming, it may be helpful to seek support from a mental health professional or a trusted friend or family member.

Wall off Calories

It is not possible to "wall off" calories or prevent them from being absorbed by the body. All calories that are consumed through food and beverages are absorbed and used by the body in some way.

If you are trying to manage your weight or maintain a healthy diet, there are several strategies you can try:

Eat a balanced diet: Focus on eating a variety of nutritious foods, including fruits, vegetables, whole grains, and lean proteins.

Watch portion sizes: Pay attention to the amount of food you are eating, and aim to control portion sizes by using smaller plates and bowls and measuring out serving sizes.

Choose foods with fewer calories: Opt for foods that are lower in calories, such as fruits and vegetables, and limit foods and beverages that are high in added sugars and unhealthy fats.

Get regular physical activity: Exercise can help burn calories and improve overall health. Aim for at least 150 minutes of moderate-intensity aerobic activity per week.

Practice mindful eating: Pay attention to your body's hunger and fullness cues, and stop eating when you feel satisfied, rather than stuffed.

By making these changes and adopting a healthy lifestyle, you can manage your weight and support overall health and well-being.